Lab Values

82 Must Know Lab Values for
Nurses. Easily Pass the
NCLEX with Practice
Questions & Rationales
Included for NCLEX Lab
Values Test Success

Eva Regan

ISBN: 1532920903
ISBN-13: 978-1532920905

Contents

Section 1: Introduction

For the vast majority of patients, laboratory test results (lab values) are assessed to make crucial decisions about their care and management. As a nurse, you will often be the first to make an assessment of a patient's lab values – it will be your responsibility to identify any values that are abnormal. Because of this, it is essential that you are aware of the normal lab value ranges in order to allow you to make well-informed assessments.

Although many find it challenging to recall the variety of common lab values, nursing students always find it effective to have a concise breakdown to hand that they can continuously revisit to make remembering critical lab values a complete breeze! This is the guide that will provide you with that concise breakdown, ensuring that you are well prepared for *all* questions related to lab values in your NCLEX exam.

The questions in your NCLEX exam will test your ability to recognize whether particular lab values are normal or abnormal. On top of this, you will need to think critically about the lab values in relation to the potential impacts on the patient. It is important to remember, however, that in reality lab value ranges may vary somewhat depending upon the equipment used for testing.

This guide provides you with a simple framework that you can apply to each lab value question – this will ensure that you are able to answer questions effectively and efficiently. For each question, you firstly need to take note of the disorder that is highlighted in the question. You will then also need to recognize which organs are impacted due to the disorder, which will guide you in selecting the correct answer to the question. For example, if the question involves a patient receiving chemotherapy who has a low white blood cell count, they will have a weakened immune system that could put them at risk of infection. By observing the lab values, you will be able to select the most appropriate preventative intervention for the client.

The list of subtopics can be seen on the contents page. Smart study strategies are outlined in the penultimate section of this guide - this will put you on a steady path to achieving success on your NCLEX exam!

Remember that ambition is the first step to success. The second step is action – hard work and determination. Purchasing this guide is an indication of your ambition, now it's time to get to work!

Best wishes,

Eva Regan

Section 2: The Components of Blood & Obtaining Samples

Blood Fundamentals

As most values are assessed via a blood samples, let's start by reviewing the basics of blood and its composition.

- **Blood**: The liquid that is pumped through the arteries, veins and capillaries by the heart. It is made up of plasma, formed elements, along with other cells types that have a variety of functions.
- **Blood Cells**: Consist of red blood cells (erythrocytes), white blood cells (leukocytes), and platelets (thrombocytes).
- **Blood Plasma**: The straw colored liquid part of the blood where blood cells are held in suspension. Composed of waters, protein, electrolytes, glucose fats, gases, and bilirubin. Plasma is crucial for the role of circulating the cellular components of the blood.
- **Blood Serum**: Thin and clear fluid that is present after coagulation. It does not contain any blood cells, fibrinogen, or platelets.

Composition of the Blood

Blood makes up approximately 8% of total body weight. Below is a concise summary of what the blood is made up of in approximate percentages.

Plasma (55% of total)

Plasma is composed of:

Proteins (7%): Albumins 54%, Globulins 38%, Fibrinogen 4%, Prothrombin 1%

Water (91%)

Solutes (2%): Ions, Nutrients, Waste products, Gases, Regulatory substances

Formed elements (45% of total)

Composed of:

Platelets: 150,000 to 400,000

Leukocytes: 4,500 to 11,000. Made up of: Neutrophils 60-70%, Lymphocytes 20-25%, Monocytes 3-8%, Eosinophils 2-4%, Basophils 0.5-1%

Erythrocytes: 4-6.2 million

Obtaining a Blood Sample

Now that you have refreshed your knowledge on the fundamental characteristics of blood, it's time to refresh yourself with the step-by-step process of obtaining blood samples from a client.

1. The nurse will check the physician's lab test prescription and then prepare the client for the test.
2. The nurse should identify any factors that could affect the test results, for example: food and medication.

3. The nurse will then clearly explain the procedure to the client, along with the reasoning for taking the sample.

4. The blood sample is drawn.

5. Pressure is immediately applied to the site of the venipuncture, followed appropriate dressing.

6. The nurse then sends the specimen to the laboratory and will take note of any specifics.

It's important to note that the nurse will always comply with standard/transmission-based precautions whilst performing the procedure of obtaining a blood sample.

Lab Value Abbreviations

As a nurse, you will encounter a number of abbreviations that are used for lab value measurements. Below is a summary of meanings for common measurement abbreviations. Try your best to familiarize yourself with these as best as you can.

- **g/dL** - Grams per deciliter
- **IU/L** - International units per liter
- **mcg/dL** - Micrograms per deciliter
- **mcg/mL** - Micrograms per milliliter
- **mEq/L** - Milliequivalents per liter
- **mg/dL** - Milligrams per deciliter
- **microunits/mL** - Microunits per milliliter
- **mL/kg** - Milliliters per kilogram

- **mm3** - Millimeters cubed
- **mm/hr** - Millimeters per hour
- **ng/mL** - Nanograms per milliliter
- **pg/mL** - Picogram per milliliter
- **units/L** - Units per liter
- **mL** - Microliters

Now that you have had a refresh on the fundamentals of blood and how it is obtained and measured, in the next section we will jump right into the different types of lab values that you will need to know in order to be successful in your NCLEX exam.

Section 3: Electrolytes

Electrolytes are minerals that are found in the blood that are made up of dissolved salts. They play a role in keeping an appropriate water balance, along with stabilizing the pH (acidity) levels in blood. To achieve this, electrolytes assist with the transport of nutrients into cells and remove waste out of cells.

Electrolyte tests are used for the identification of electrolyte (salt) imbalances. **Sodium** and **potassium** are the most common electrolytes that are assessed, but other electrolytes such as **chloride** and **bicarbonate** can also be monitored. Electrolyte tests are commonly used when there is suspicion of high blood pressure, kidney disease, and heart failure. On top of this, electrolyte levels may be monitored if a client has been prescribed medications such as ACE inhibitors and diuretics.

Below you will find a summary of each electrolyte, along with the normal adult electrolyte lab values that you need to know.

Sodium

Normal Adult Value: **135 to 145 mEq/L**

Key Points

- Sodium is a major cation (positively charged ion) within extracellular fluid.
- It helps to sustain osmotic pressure, along with acid-base balance.
- Nerve impulse transmission is aided by sodium.
- The small intestine absorbs sodium and it is expelled by urine.
- 15 mEq is the minimum daily requirement for sodium.

Potassium

Normal Adult Value: **3.5-5.1 mEq/L**

Key Points

- Potassium is a major intracellular cation.
- Controls cellular water balance.
- Regulates muscle cell electrical conduction, along with acid-base balance.
- Potassium is received through diet and is conserved or expelled depending on cellular requirements by the kidney.
- Uses of potassium level assessment: cardiovascular function, renal function, and gastrointestinal function.
- Potassium can also be used to indicate whether IV replacement therapy is needed.

- **Note:** Elevated levels of white blood cell count and platelet counts can produce potassium levels that are falsely elevated in lab values.

Chloride

Normal Adult Value: **98 to 107 mEq/L**

Key Points

- A hydrochloric acid salt that supports the balance of fluid both inside and outside of cells.
- The most common extracellular body anion.
- Plays the role of offsetting cations (e.g. sodium).
- Helps with blood volume, blood pressure, acid-base balance, digestion, water balance, and osmotic pressure.
- **Note:** Diarrhea and/or vomiting will affect levels of chloride in lab values.

Bicarbonate

Normal Adult Value: **22 to 29 mEq/L**

Key Points

- Part of the carbonic acid/bicarbonate buffer.

- Regulates pH levels of body fluids.
- **Note:** The consumption of acidic solutions can produce increased values, and the consumption of alkaline solutions can produce decreased values.

Section 4: Coagulation Tests

Coagulation tests are used to measure the blood's ability to clot and the amount of time it takes to clot. It is important that you have a good understanding of the different tests that are used, along with the normal lab values for each one.

Activated Partial Thromboplastin Time (APTT)

Normal Value for Test: **20 to 36 Seconds (Dependent on Activator Type)**

Key Points

- By measuring the time it takes recalcified citrated plasma to clot after partial thromboplastin is added to it, APTT assesses the functioning of the coagulation sequence.
- Apart from VII and XIII, deficiencies and inhibitors of all factors are screened for.
- Used to screen for coagulation disorders.
- Generally used to assess heparin therapy.
  Notes:

- Samples should not be drawn from an arm where heparin is being infused.
- Specimens should be transported to the laboratory as soon as possible.

- When a patient is receiving heparin, the APTT should be 1.5 to 2.5 higher than normal.
- Bleeding precautions should be taken if the APTT value is prolonged beyond 90 seconds.

Prothrombin Time (PT) and International Normalized Ratio (INR)

Normal Values for Tests:

Prothrombin Time (PT)

Adult Male: 9.6 to 11.8 Seconds

Adult Female: 9.5 to 11.3 Seconds.

International Normalized Ratio (INR)

For Standard Warfarin Therapy: 2 to 3.

For High-Dose Warfarin Therapy: 3 to 4.5.

Key Points

- Prothrombin: A glycoprotein that is vitamin K dependent and is produced by the liver. It is essential for the formation of fibrin clots.
- Depending on the PT method used by the laboratory, a normal or control value is established.
  PT test evaluates:

- The time (in seconds) it takes for the formation of clots.
- Monitors warfarin sodium therapy response.
- Dysfunction of the extrinsic clotting system that results from liver disease, disseminated intravascular coagulation, or deficiency in vitamin K.
- *A PT value that is **plus or minus 2 seconds from the control value** is considered normal.*
  INR measures:

- Evaluates oral anticoagulant effects.
- The INR is calculated by raising the PR ratio to the power of the international sensitivity index in correspondence to the throboplastin reagent that is used.
  Notes:

- Before anticoagulation therapy, a baseline PT should be drawn.
- If warfarin therapy is concurrent with heparin therapy, this could increase the PT up to 5 hours.
- PT can be decreased due to consumption of green leafy vegetables that elevate the amount of vitamin K that is absorbed.
- Anticoagulation therapy that is orally administered will generally keep the PT value at 1.5 - 2 times the lab value.
- A PT value that is longer than 30 seconds, bleeding precautions should be taken.

Clotting Time Test

Normal Value: **8 to 15 minutes**

Key Points

- Measures the time it takes for all factors to interact in process of clotting.
  Notes:

- Results are affected by heparin therapy, therefore for the patient should not have heparin therapy 3 before the collection of a specimen.
- Anticoagulant therapy will incorrectly prolong the test results.

Platelet Count Test

Normal Value: **150,000 to 400,000 cells/mm3**

Key Points

- Platelets act by forming hemostatic plugs, retracting clots, activate coagulation factors.
- The bone marrow produces platelets that act in hemostasis.
  Notes:

- Patients with thrombocytopenia should be carefully monitored for bleeding.
- Platelet counts can be elevated by cold weather and physical activity.
- For patients with a low blood count, bleeding precautions should be taken.

Section 5: Erythrocyte Tests

Erythrocyte or red blood cell tests are used for the diagnosis and assessment of a number of infections and diseases. Here is a summary of the most common tests, along with their normal values.

Erythrocyte Sedimentation Rate (ESR)

Normal Value: **0 to 30 mm/hr, depending on client's age.**

Key Points

- Assesses illnesses that are linked with inflammation, acute and chronic infections, cancers, and autoimmune diseases.
- Fasting is not required for ESR.

Hemoglobin and Hematocrit

Normal Values:

Hemoglobin

Adult Male: 14 to 16.5 g/dL

Female Adult: 12 to 15 g/dL

Hematocrit

Adult Male: 42% to 52%

Adult Female: 35% to 47%

Key Points

Hemoglobin:

- Key component of erythrocytes.
- Transports oxygen and carbon dioxide.
- A key factor in determining and identifying anemia.
Hematocrit:

- Represents the mass of red blood cells.
- Key factor in identifying anemia or polycythemia.
- Fasting is not necessary.

Iron

Normal Values:

Adult Male: 65 to 175 mcg/dL

Adult Female: 50 to 170 mcg/dL

Key Points

- Found in hemoglobin.
- Carries oxygen from the lungs to tissues.
- Assists the return of carbon dioxide to the lungs.
- A factor in the diagnosis of anemia and hemolytic disorders.
  Notes:

- Iron level will be elevated if the patient has ingested prior to the test.

Red Blood Cell Count (Erythrocytes)

Normal Values:

Adult Male: 4.5 to 6.2 million/mL

Adult Female: 4 to 5.5 million/mL

Key Points

- Acts in the transportation of hemoglobin – delivering oxygen to the tissues of the body.
- Red bone marrow forms red blood cells and they have a 120-day life span.
- Red blood cells are taken out of the blood by the liver, spleen, and bone marrow.
- Assists in the diagnosis of anemias.
- Fasting is not necessary for red blood cell count testing.

Section 6: Serum Enzymes and Cardiac Markers

<u>Creatine Kinase (CK)</u>

Normal Values: **26-174 units/L**

Key Points

- An enzyme that is found in muscle tissue and brain tissue.
- Indicates tissue catabolism that results from cell trauma.
- Creatine Kinase will start to rise within 6 hours following damage to muscles, and will reach a maximum level at approx. 18 hours after muscle damage.
- Levels return to a normal level within 2/3 days following the damage.
- Creatine Kinase testing is used to identify myocardial damage, skeletal muscle damage, and damage to the central nervous system.
- The isoenzymes of creatine kinase are made up of CK-MB (found in cardiac muscle), CK-BB (found in the brain tissue), and CK-MM (found in skeletal muscles).

<u>CK Isoenzymes Normal Levels:</u>

CK-MB: 0%-5% of total

CK-MM: 95%-100% of total

CK-BB: 0%

Notes:

- Vigorous activity should be avoided for 24 prior to testing if the test is assessing skeletal muscle.
- The patient should avoid alcohol for 24 hours prior to testing.
- Creating Kinase can be falsely elevated by injections and any procedures that are invasive.

Lactate Dehydrogenase (LDH)

Normal Values: **140-280 units/L**

Key Points

- Myocardial infarctions affect the LDH isoenzymes LDH1 and LDH2.
- Lactate Dehydrogenase (LDH) levels elevate approx. 24 hours following myocardial infarction and reach a maximum at approx. 48-72 hours.
- Levels generally return to normal with 1 to 2 weeks.
- When LDH1 is higher than LDH2, this assists the diagnosis of myocardial infarction.
Notes:

- Tests should be repeated across 3 days in a row.

Normal Levels of LDH Isoenzymes

LDH1: 14% to 26%

LDH2: 29% to 39%

LDH3: 20% to 26%

LDH4: 8% to 16%

LDH5: 6% to 16%

Troponins

Normal Values:

Troponin I: Below 0.6 ng/mL.

Troponin I Higher Than 1.5 ng/mL: Indicates Myocardial Infarction.

Troponin T Higher Than 0.1-0.2 ng/mL: Indicates Myocardial Infarction

Key Points

- Regulatory protein that is in striated muscle.
- Elevated troponins occur when there is myocardium damage as a result of infarction.
- The levels generally increase within 3 hours of the injury.

- Troponin I levels may remain increased for up to 10 days.
- Troponin T levels may remain increased for up to 14 days.
- Consecutive measurements are essential in order to compare initial baseline levels.
  Notes:

- Testing should be repeated each day for 3-5 days.

Myoglobin

Normal Values: **Below 90 mcg/L**

An elevation can be an indication of myocardial infarction.

Key Points

- Oxygen-binding protein found in striated muscle.
- Skeletal muscle injury will result in myoglobin being released into the blood.
- Levels can elevate within 2 hours of myocardial infarction, and quickly fall after approx. 7 hours.
  Notes:

Natriuretic Peptides

Normal Values:

ANP: 22 to 27 pg/mL

BNP: Below 100 pg/mL

CNP: N/A

Key Points

- Neuroendocrine peptides that are utilized for the identification of congestive heart failure.
  3 types of peptides:

- Atrial Natriuretic Peptides (ANP) (produced in the cardiac atrial muscle)
- Brain natriuretic Peptides (BNP) (produced in the cardiac ventricle muscle)
- C-type Natriuretic Peptides (CNP) (produced by the endothelial cells)
- BNP is the central marker for the identification of congestive heart failure with dyspnea.
  Notes:

- The larger the elevation of the level of BNP, the more serious the congestive heart failure.
- An elevated BNP level indicates dyspnea from congestive heart failure, a normal BNP level indicates a pulmonary complication due to congestive heart failure.

Section 7: Gastrointestinal Tests

Albumin

Normal Value: **3.4 to 5 g/dL**

Key Points

- A key plasma protein in the blood.
- Albumin sustains oncotic pressure and provides transportation for bilirubin, medications, fatty acids, hormones, and other water insoluble substances.
- Albumin is elevated during dehydration and diarrhea.
- Albumin is decreased in acute infections, alcoholism, and ascites.
- If albumin is detected in urine, it is an indication of the renal functioning abnormally.
- Fasting is not necessary for albumin testing.

Alkaline Phosphatase

Normal Value: **4.5 to 13 King-Armstrong units/dL**

Key Points

- Enzyme that is found in the liver, bone, and intestine.
- Alkaline Phosphatase level rises during the growth of bones, liver disease, and obstruction of the bile duct.

Notes:

- Fasting may be necessary 12 hours prior to the test.
- Hepatotoxic medications can falsely elevate levels

Ammonia

Normal Value: **10 to 80 mcg/dL**

Key Points

- A consequence of protein catabolism.
- Mostly produced by bacteria in the gut acting on proteins.
- The liver metabolizes ammonia and is expelled as urea by the kidneys.
- Hepatic dysfunction can cause elevated ammonia levels which is an indication of hepatic coma.
  Notes:

- The patient must fast (apart from water) for 8-10 hours prior to the test.
- Smoking should also be avoided for 10 hours before the test.

Alanine Aminotransferase (ALT)

Normal Value: **4 to 6 International Units/L**

Key Points

- ALT is utilized for the identification of liver hepatocellular disease and to assess the extent to which it deteriorates.
  Notes:

- Elevated levels may be caused by prior intramuscular injections.
- Fasting is unnecessary.

Aspartate Aminotransferase (AST)

Normal Value: **0 to 35 units/L**

Key Points

- Test is used to assess a patient that is suspected to have hepatocellular disease.
- Can also be used with cardiac markers to assess evaluate coronary artery occlusive disease.
  Notes:

- Elevated levels may be caused by prior intramuscular injections.
- Fasting is unnecessary.

Amylase

Key Points

- Created by the pancreas and salivary glands.
- Assists complex carbohydrate digestion and is expelled by the kidneys.
- After 3-6 hours following the onset of acute pancreatitis, levels of amylase slightly rise.
- The level reaches a maximum approx. 24 hours after the onset, and returns to normal after 2-3 days.
  Notes:

- A number of medications can cause a false/positive result.

Lipase

Normal Value: **10 to 140 units/L**

Key Point

- A pancreatic enzyme that converts triglycerides and fats into glycerol and fatty acids.
- Pancreatic disorders cause elevated levels of lipase – generally 2-3 days after the onset.
- Levels can remain elevated for 2 weeks.
  Notes:

- Lipase activity can be increased by Endoscopic

Retrograde Cholangiopancreatography (ERCP)

Bilirubin

Direct Bilirubin: 0 to 0.3 mg/dL

Indirect Bilirubin: 0.1 to1 mg/dL

Total Bilirubin: Below 1.5 mg/dL

Key Points

- Created by the liver, bone marrow, and spleen.
- Also results from hemoglobin breakdown.
- Direct bilirubin is split down into direct bilirubin (excreted through the intestinal tract).
- Indirect Bilirubin is circulates in the bloodstream.
- Total levels are elevated with jaundice, and the direct and indirect levels are used to identify the jaundice cause.
  Notes:

- Client should eat a diet that contains few yellow foods approx. 4 days prior to testing.
- Fasting is required 4 hours prior to the drawing of blood.
- Elevated results will occur due to alcohol, morphine sulfate, aspirin, and Vitamin C.

Lipids

Cholesterol: 140 to 199 mg/dL

Low-Density Lipoproteins: Below 130mg/dL

HDLs: 30 to 70 mg/dL

Triglycerides: Below 200 mg/dL

Key Points

- Lipids in the blood consist of cholesterol, phospholipids, and triglycerides.
- The assessment of lipids is made up of:
- Cholesterol High-Density Lipoprotein (HDL)
- Low-Density Lipoprotein (LDL)
- Triglycerides

- Chloesterol is found in all tissues of the body – it is a main component of LDLs, cell membranes, and brain and nerve cells.
- Triglycerides make up small part of LDLs, but a key part of very low-density lipoproteins. They are synthesized from protein, fatty acids, and glucose, and are taken in through the diet.
- Elevated LDL, cholesterol, and triglyceride levels put the patient at risk of coronary artery disease.
- HDL assists in the protection against coronary artery disease risk.
  Notes:

- Lipid levels can be increased by oral contraceptives.

- The patient must fast (apart from water) for 13-24 hours prior to testing, along with no intake of alcohol for 24 hours before testing.

Protein

Normal Value: **6 to 8 g/dL**

Key Points

- A representation of the total amounts of albumin and globulins within the plasma
- Controls osmotic pressure and essential for hormone formation, enzyme formation, and antibody formation.
- Levels of protein are increased in autoimmune collagen disorders, Addison's disease, Crohn's disease, chronic infection.
- Levels of protein are decreased in cirrhosis, burns, edema, and hepatic disease.
  Notes:

- The patient should avoid fatty foods for 8 hours prior to testing.

Uric Acid

Normal Values:

Adult Male: 4.5 to 8 mg/dL

Adult Female: 2.5 to 6.2 mg/dL

Key Points

- Created as guanine and purines adenine are metabolized during the creation and degradation of RNA and DNA.
- Created as a result of dietary purines metabolism.
- Increased levels of uric acid deposits in the soft tissue and joints cause gout.
- Hyperuricemia may be caused by slowed renal excretion of uric acid increased cellular turnover.
- Increased levels pose risk for urate stones in the kidney.
  Notes:

- The patient should fast for 8 hours prior to testing.
- Results may be falsely increased by caffeine, theophylline, and vitamin C.

Section 8: Glucose Tests

Blood glucose tests are generally used for the identification of hyperglycemia (high blood glucose) and hypoglycemia (low blood glucose). They are also used to screen patients for diabetes.

Fasting Blood Glucose

Normal Value: **70 to 110 mg/dL**

Key Points

- Created in the digestion of carbohydrate digestion and glycogen conversion by the liver.
- The key energy source of the body's cellular energy.
- Vital for erythrocyte and brain functioning.
- Fasting blood glucose levels are used in the diagnosis of hypoglycemia and diabetes.
  Notes:

- Fasting is requires for 8 to 12 hours prior to testing.
- Patients with diabetes should refrain from insulin medication until after testing.

Glucose Tolerance Test

Normal Values:

Glucose Tolerance Test (Oral)

Baseline fasting: 70 to 110 mg/dL

30-min fasting: 110 to 170 mg/dL

60-min fasting: 120 to 170 mg/dL

90-min fasting: 100 to 140 mg/dL

120-min fasting: 70 to 120 mg/dL

Key Points

- Helps in the diagnosis of diabetes mellitus.
- Diabetes is indicated if glucose levels reach higher than normal levels at the 1 and 2 hour intervals after ingestion or injection of glucose, and if levels take longer than usual to return to the fasting level. **Notes:**

- The patient should consume a high amount of carbohydrates 3 days prior to testing.
- The patient should fast for 10 to 16 hours prior to testing.
- The patient should refrain from smoking, alcohol, and caffeine for 36 hours prior to testing.
- The patient should refrain from physical exercise 8 hours before and following testing.
- Patients with diabetes should refrain from insulin medication until after testing.

Glycosylated Hemoglobin

Normal Values *(As a Percentage of Total Hemoglobin):*

Good Diabetes Control: 7% or Below

Fair Diabetes Control: 7% to 8%

Poor Diabetes Control: Large Than 8%

Key Points

- Glycosylated hemoglobin (HbA1c) is hemoglobin to which glucose is bound.
- Glycosylated hemoglobin is an indication of the extent to which glucose levels have been regulated in the previous 3-4 months.
- An increase in HbA1c is usually caused by hyperglycemia in patients with diabetes.
  Notes:

- Fasting is unnecessary.

Glycosylated Serum Albumin (Fructosamine)

Normal Values:

Patient Without Diabetes: 1.5 to 2.7 mmol/L

Patient With Diabetes: 2 to 5 mmol/L

Key Points

- Glycosylated Serum Albumin is a representation of the average levels of serum glucose over a 2-3 week time period.
- It is more sensitive to changes than glycosylated hemoglobin.
  Notes:

- Fasting is required 12 hours prior to testing.

Diabetes Mellitus Autoantibody Panel

Normal Values: **Below 1:4 Titer Without Antibody Detected**

Key Points:

- Testing is used for the evaluation of resistance to insulin, the identification of type 1 diabetes, and the detection of insulin allergy.
  Notes:

- Fasting before testing is not required.

Section 9: Renal Function Tests

Both creatinine and urea nitrogen levels should be evaluated when renal function is assessed. Below are the normal values for these tests.

Creatinine

Normal Value: **0.6 to 1.3 mg/dL**

Key Points

- An indication of renal function.
- A slowing of the glomerular filtration rate is indicated by elevated levels of creatinine.
  Notes:

- Vigorous exercise should be avoided for 8 hours.

Blood Urea Nitrogen

Normal Value: **8 to 25 mg/dL**

Key Points

- The nitrogen part of urea that is created in the liver through the breakdown of enzymatic protein.

- Increased levels indicate a decrease in the glomerular filtration rate.

Section 10: Elements

Calcium

Normal Value: **8.6 to 10 mg/dL**

Key Points

- A cation that is absorbed into the blood as a result of intake in the diet.
- Serves the formation of bones, the transmission of nerve impulses, and myocardial and skeletal muscle contraction.
- Calcium converts prothrombin to thrombin which helps blood clotting.
  Notes:

- Fasting could be necessary for 8 hours prior to testing.
- Normal levels of calcium should be consumed prior to testing, approx. 800mg per day.

Magnesium

Normal Value: **1.6 to 2.6 mg/dL**

Key Points

- Determines renal function and metabolic activity.
- Essential in the blood clotting process.
- Controls neuromuscular activity.
- Affects the metabolism of calcium.
  Notes:

- Levels increase as a result of ongoing use of magnesium products.
- Large amounts of body fluid loss will decrease magnesium levels.

Phosphorus

Normal Value: **2.7 to 4.5 mg/dL**

Key Points

- Essential for the formation of bones, the storage and release of energy, the metabolism of carbohydrates, and urinary acid-base balance.
- Taken in from food and expelled by the kidneys.
- Large volumes of phosphorus are found in skeletal muscles and bones.
  Notes:

- Fasting is required before testing.

Section 11: Thyroid Tests

Normal Values:

Thyroid-Stimulating Hormone (Thyrotropin): 0.2 to 5.4 microunits/mL

Thyroxine (T4): 5 to 12 mcg/dL

Thyroxine, free (FT4): 0.8 to 2.4 ng/dL

Triiodothyronine (T3): 80 to 230 ng/dL

Key Points:

- Thyroid tests are used when there is suspicion of a thyroid disorder.
- Assists in distinguishing between primary thyroid disease and causes that are secondary and irregularities in levels of thyroxine-binding globulin.
  Notes:

- If the patient has had a radionuclide scan within 7 days prior to testing, this can invalidate the test results.

Section 12: White Blood Cell Count

Normal Value: **4500 to 11,000 cells/mm3**

Neutrophils: 1800 to 7800 cells/mm3

Bands: 0 to 700 cells/mm3

Eosinophils: 0 to 450 cells/mm3

Basophils: 0 to 200 cells/mm3

Lymphocytes: 1000 to 4800 cells/mm3

Monocytes: 0 to 800 cells/mm3

Key Points

- White blood cells work in the body's immune defense system.
- The assessment of leukocyte distribution is indicated by the white blood cell count.
  Notes:

- An elevated level of immature neutrophils in the blood is referred to as a 'shift to the left.
- A low white blood cell count indicates depression of bone marrow or an infection with an overwhelming demand for neutrophils.

- A high white blood cell count combined with a shit to the left indicates a response to a severe infection or inflammation.
- When cells have an unusually high level of nuclear segments, this is referred to as a 'shift to the right. E.g. this is found in liver disease and Down syndrome.

Section 13: Hepatitis and HIV

Hepatitis
Values for Detection:

Hepatitis A:

- Immunoglobulin M (IgM) Antibody to hepatitis A virus.

- Total Antibody to Hepatitis A virus.

Hepatitis B:

- Presence of hepatitis B core antigen (HBcAg), surface antigen (HBsAg), envelope antigen (HBeAg).

Hepatitis C:

- Antibodies to hepatitis C virus.

Serological Hepatitis D:

- Hepatitis D antigen (HDAg) in the early stages of infection.

- Presence of anti–hepatitis D virus antibody.

Serological Hepatitis E:

- IgM and IgG antibodies to hepatitis E

Hepatitus G:

Can be found in donors of blood, hemodialysis patients, IV drug users.

Key Points:

- Testing for hepatitis includes radioimmunoassay, microparticle enzyme immunoassay, Enzyme-linked Immunosorbent Assay (ELISA).
- To define the type of hepatitis, serological tests for hepatitis virus markers are used.

HIV

Values for Detection:

- Positive Western blot or IFA

- A negative ELISA test should be repeated in 3-6 months.

Key Points:

- The detection of HIV that causes AIDS.

- Enzyme-linked Immunosorbent Assay (ELISA), immunofluorescence assay (IFA), and Western blot are tests that are used to detect HIV.
- ELISA tests need to be repeated, and if reactive Western blot or IFA should be used as a follow up test.

CD4+ T-Cell Test Counts

- The number of CD4+ T-cell count generally increases as HIV progresses.

Normal CD4+ T-Cell Count: Between 500 and 1600 cells/L

Problems with immune system: When T cell count is between 200 and 499 cells/L

Serious problems with immune system: When T cell count is below 200 cells/L

CD4-to-CD8 Ratio

- Assesses the progression of HIV.
- A ratio of approx. 2:1 is normal.
- **Viral culture:** placing the blood cells of the infected patient in a culture medium and the assessing the amount of reverse transcriptase activity.

- **Viral load testing:** Evaluating whether HIV genetic material (RNA) is present in the patient's blood.

P24 Antigen Assay

- Evaluates the amount of HIV viral core protein in the patient's serum.

Oral HIV Testing

- A device is positioned against the cheek and the gum of the client.
- Fluid is taken into an absorbable pad.
- The fluid in a HIV positive patient will contain antibodies.
- If the test result is positive, a blood test is required for a confirmation of the results.

Home HIV Test Kits

- A drop of blood is put on a card for testing.
- The card is sent to a laboratory that conducts testing for the presence of antibodies.

Section 14: Normal Urine Tests & Therapeutic Medication Levels

Urine Tests - Name of Test & Value

- Color: Pale yellow
- Odor: Aromatic odor, comparable to ammonia
- Turbidity: Clear
- pH Level: 4.5 to 7.8
- Specific gravity: 1.016 to 1.022
- Glucose: Below 0.5 g/day
- Ketones: None
- Protein: None
- Bilirubin: None
- Casts: None to few
- Crystals: None
- Bacteria: None or Below 1000/mL
- Red blood cells: Below 3 cells/HPF
- White blood cells: Equal to or below 4 cells/HPF
- Chloride: 110 to 250 mEq/24 hours
- Magnesium: 7.3 to 12.2 mg/dL
- Potassium: 25 to 125 mEq/24 hours
- Sodium: 40 to 220 mEq/24 hours
- Uric acid: 250 to 750 mg/24 hours

Theraputic Medication Levels

- Acetaminophen (Tylenol): 10 to 20 mcg/mL
- Amikacin (Amikin): 25 to 30 mcg/mL
- Amitriptyline: 120 to 150 ng/mL
- Carbamazepine (Tegretol): 5 to 12 mcg/mL

- <u>Chloramphenicol (Chloromycetin):</u> 10 to 20 mcg/mL
- <u>Desipramine (Norpramin):</u> 150 to 300 ng/mL
- <u>Digoxin (Lanoxin):</u> 0.5 to 2 ng/mL
- <u>Disopyramide (Norpace):</u> 2 to 5 mcg/mL
- <u>Ethosuximide (Zarontin):</u> 40 to 100 mcg/mL
- <u>Gentamicin:</u> 5 to 10 mcg/mL
- <u>Imipramine (Tofranil):</u> 150 to 300 ng/mL
- <u>Lidocaine (Xylocaine):</u> 1.5 to 5 mcg/mL
- <u>Lithium (Lithobid):</u> 0.5 to 1.2 mEq/L
- <u>Magnesium sulfate:</u> 4 to 7 mg/dL
- <u>Phenobarbital (Luminal):</u> 10 to 30 mcg/mL
- <u>Phenytoin (Dilantin):</u> 10 to 20 mcg/mL
- <u>Propranolol (Inderal):</u> 50 to 100 ng/mL
- <u>Salicylate:</u> 100 to 250 mcg/mL
- <u>Theophylline:</u> 10 to 20 mcg/mL
- <u>Tobramycin (Nebcin):</u> 5 to 10 mcg/mL
- <u>Valproic acid (Depakene):</u> 50 to 100 mcg/mL

Section 15: Practice Questions and Rationales

1. A patient who has atrial fibrillation is having maintenance therapy of warfarin sodium (Coumadin) and they have a 35 second prothrombin time (PT). What type of prescription should the nurse expect based on the prothrombin time?

A. An additional dose of heparin sodium

B. Preventing the next warfarin dose

C. Increasing the next warfarin dose

D. Administering the next warfarin dose

Answer A is correct. In an adult male the normal PT is 9.6-11.8 seconds, and in a female adult the normal PT is 9.5-11.3 seconds. A PT level that is 1.5 to 2 times larger than the normal level is a therapeutic PT level. A PT of 35 seconds is high and therefore further doses would not be expected. Answers A, C, and D are incorrect because these would not be prescriptions that would be anticipated.

Test Tip: Remember that a 30 second or higher PT will mean the patient is at risk of bleeding.

2. A 2.4 ng/mL serum digoxin result is observed for a test that was taken from a patient earlier in the day. Which of the following actions should the nurse take immediately?

A. Inform the physician.

B. Evaluate the patient's last pulse rate.

C. Record the normal value on the patient's flow sheet.

D. Provide the next dose of medication.

Answer A is correct. 0.5-2 ng/mL is the normal therapeutic range for digoxin. 2.4 ng/mL is greater than the normal therapeutic range, therefore this is an indication of toxicity. Because of this, the physician should be informed who may arrange holding further digoxin with additional prescriptions. Answer C is incorrect because this is an abnormal level. Answer D is incorrect because the next does should not be given at this level. Answer B is incorrect because checking the pulse rate of the patient is inappropriate in this circumstance.

Test Tip: Be sure to remember the therapeutic range – if the value falls outside the range, immediate intervention is needed.

3. A patient with a urinary tract infection and dehydration has been admitted to the hospital. What level of blood urea nitrogen level will indicate to the nurse that the patient has received adequate volume?

A. 3 mg/dL

B. 15 mg/dL

C. 29 mg/dL

D. 35 mg/dL

Answer B is correct. A blood nitrogen level of 8 to 25 mg/dL is the normal range. Answer B is incorrect because this is a level that is below the normal value – this may happen with fluid volume overload. Answers C and D are incorrect because they are an indication of ongoing dehydration.

Test tip: Try to use a process of elimination in order to direct yourself to the correct answer.

4. A patient in the emergency room is reporting chest pain that started a few hours earlier. A 0.6 ng/mL level of

troponin T is found from a blood specimen. What does this result indicate?

A. Normal level

B. Low value that is an indication of possible gastritis

C. A level that is an indication of a myocardial infarction

D. A level that is an indication of possible angina

Answer C is correct. Troponin is found in striated muscle and is a regulatory protein. Elevated amounts of troponin are released into the blood when there is damage to the myocardium as a result of an infarction. Myocardial infarction is indicated by a troponin T level above 0.1-0.2 ng/mL.

5. In order to treat a deep vein thrombosis, a patient is receiving a continuous heparin sodium intravenous infusion. The patient has an activated partial thromboplastin (aPTT) time of 65 seconds. Which of the following actions does the nurse expect to be required?

A. Stopping the heparin infusion

B. Increasing the heparin infusion rate

3. Decreasing the heparin infusion rate

4. Maintaining the heparin infusion at the same rate

Answer D is correct. The normal APTT is 20 to 26 seconds. This depends on the activator that is used for testing. In deep vein thrombosis, the therapeutic does of APTT is 1.5 to 2.5 times normal. Therefore, the patient's should not be below 30 seconds or above 90 seconds. In this situation, the patient's APTT is in the therapeutic range, therefore the heparin infusion should be kept at the same rate.

6. A morning dose of furosemide (Lasix) is due for a patient that has a history of cardiovascular disease. Before administering furosemide, what level of serum potassium should be reported?

A. 3.2 mEq/L

B. 3.8 mEq/L

C. 4.2 mEq/L

D. 4.8 mEq/L

Answer A is correct. 3.5 to 5.1 mEq/L is the normal level of serum potassium in an adult. 3.2 mEq/L is below the therapeutic range – the administration of furosemide to a patient with a history of cardiac disease and low potassium can lead to ventricular dysrhythmias. Answers B, C, and D are incorrect because they are in the normal range.

Test tip: Remember the normal potassium level and look for the abnormal level.

7. A platelet count of 300,000 cells/mm3 is reported for a patient that has a history of gastrointestinal bleeding. What should the nurse do after seeing the results from the laboratory?

A. Report the count as abnormally low.

B. Report the count as abnormally high.

C. Place the patient on bleeding precautions.

D. Place the normal report in the patient's medical record.

Answer D is correct. The normal range for a platelet count is 150,00 to 400,000 cells/mm3, therefore the nurse should place the normal report in the patient's record. Answers A, B, and C are incorrect because the level is not above or below the normal range, and bleeding precautions are not necessary.

8. A patient with cirrhosis has tried a diet that has both an excess and deficiency of protein, and neither of these has been helpful. The client is currently on a diet with optimal amounts of protein. Which protein level produces the most satisfactory state for the patient?

A. 0.4 g/dL

B. 3.7 g/dL

C. 6.4 g/dL

D. 9.8 g/dL

Answer C is correct. 6 to 8 g/dL is the normal range for serum protein level in an adult patient. A patient with cirrhosis generally has a low protein levels due to insufficient nutrition. Answers A and B are incorrect because they indicate values that are below the normal range. Answer D is incorrect because it indicates a value above the normal range.

9. A glycosylated hemoglobin A1c level of 9% is identified for a patient with diabetes mellitus. What should the nurse teach the patient based on this result?

A. To avoid infection.

B. Take in adequate fluids.

C. Prevent and acknowledge hypoglycemia.

D. Prevent and acknowledge hyperglycemia.

Answer D is correct. A glycosylated hemoglobin A1c level is the measurement of glucose that is permanently bound to red blood cells. A level of 7% or below is an indication of good control, 7-8% indicates control that is sufficient, higher than 8% indicates insufficient control. High levels of blood glucose will result in high levels of glycosylation. Therefore, hyperglycemia can be identified and the patient should be instructed about the prevention of hyperglycemic episodes.

10. A patient who has been diagnosed with cancer is immunosuppressed and being cared for by the nurse.

Which of the following white blood cell counts would make the nurse consider the implementation of neutropenic precautions:

A. 2000 cells/mm3

B. 5800 cells/mm3

C. 8400 cells/mm3

D. 11,000 cells/mm3

Answer A is correct. 4500-11,000/mm3 is the normal white blood cell count. A patient is immunosuppressed when they have a decrease in the amount of circulating white blood cells. The nurse should implement neutropenic precautions when the patient's count is significantly below the normal range. Answers B, C and D are incorrect because they are in the normal range.

11. A patient in the emergency room has said they have been taking twice the prescribed dose of wardarin (Coumadin) over the previous 7 days. What should the nurse prepare to do once noting that the patient has no signs of bleeding?

A. Start preparing to administer an antidote.

B. Take a sample for type and crossmatch and transfuse the client.

C. Take a sample for an activated partial thromboplastin time (aPTT) level.

D. Take a sample for prothrombin time (PT) and international normalized ratio (INR).

Answer D is correct. In order to determine the patient's anticoagulation status, the nurse should draw a PT sample and INR level. This will produce information that will indicate what will be the best treatment for the patient. For example, a blood transfusion may or an antidote such as vitamin K might be required.

12. A 45-year-old patient has been diagnosed with chronic pancreatitis. Which of the following levels does the nurse expect the patient's serum amylase to be?

A. 45 units/L

B. 100 units/L

C. 300 units/L

D. 500 units/L

Answer C is correct. 25-151 units/L is the normal range for amylase. In chronic pancreatitis, the elevation in amylase is no greater than three times the normal value. The value may be greater than five times the normal value in acute pancreatitis. Answers A and B are incorrect because they are in the normal range. Answer D is incorrect because this is a level that is consistent with acute pancreatitis.

Test tip: Make sure you are familiar with the key word 'chronic' and its associated level.

13. A hemoglobin level of 10.8 g/dL is reported for a female adult. Which of the following conditions in the patient's history is most likely to cause this value?

A. Dehydration

B. Heart failure

C. Iron deficiency anemia

D. Chronic obstructive pulmonary disease

Answer C is correct. 12-15 g/dL is the normal level of hemoglobin for an adult female. Iron deficiency anemia can produce decrease lower levels of hemoglobin. Answer A is incorrect because dehydration can result in higher levels of hemoglobin due to hemoconcentration. Answers B and D are incorrect because heart failure and chronic obstructive pulmonary disease can elevate levels of hemoglobin due to the greater need for oxygen carrying capacity by the body.

Section 16: Study and Exam Preparation Tips

Studying for the NCLEX is a daunting challenge for every nursing student. Despite this, it is completely manageable and with the right approach, and success can be guaranteed.

In preparing for the NCLEX, there are three central elements that are of most important: **understanding, organization,** and **practice.** This study guide is designed for those who already have a good understanding of nursing practice. *Sections 2-6* of the guide are simply designed to refresh your memory and help you retain essential information that you will need to answer the practice questions in *Section 7.*

In this section, we have compiled some essential review strategies that will assist you in effective preparation for the NCLEX!

<u>Study Tips:</u>

- **Learning the details comes first!**
- Before going through the questions, it is important that you have come to grasp with the content that is being tested.

- Practice questions are designed to test and further your knowledge, and to make sure you know how to answer the questions efficiently and successfully.

- **Repetition is key!**
- Memorizing is key when it comes to dealing with conversion factors, laboratory values, among other things. It is therefore useful to devote a set time each day to studying the information.

- On top of this, we encourage you to make best use of the time you spend commuting by continually going over key points.

- Repeating information just before you go to sleep also helps you memorize information you find particularly difficult to retain.

- **Test yourself!**
- As the old saying goes, practice is the key to success. The questions presented in this guide are representative of what you should expect in the NCLEX exam.

- Testing yourself is essential to knowing whether you are well prepared for the exam.

- Make sure to practice as much as possible and once you are getting closer to the actual exam, time yourself, allowing approximately one minute per question.

- **Learn from your mistakes!**
- If there are questions you haven't answered correctly, then see whether you understand the rationale and go over your revision notes again to make sure you have understood it fully.

- Make sure to test yourself again on questions that you initially answered incorrectly.

- All questions in this guide are numbered. Make sure to note down the questions you answered incorrectly and skip forward to these questions next time!

Exam Tips:

These are tips you should apply when you are sitting the exam. Try to also apply these when you are going over practice questions so it becomes second nature!

- **Read the questions carefully!**
- Being alert is key to successfully passing the NCLEX! Skimming through questions is the mistake most often made.

- It is crucial to make sure you read the question carefully and that you fully understand what it is the question is asking.

- If necessary, reword the question in your own words. This often helps in crafting an appropriate answer.

- **Look for keywords!**
- Keywords will help you work through the questions more efficiently.

- It is also advisable to avoid answers that include keywords such as all, always, every, except, must, never, no, none and only because they are rarely correct as they often limit or qualify the actual correct answer.

- **Use the method of elimination!**
- This is particularly useful if you are not straight away sure which option is the correct answer.

- Eliminate the answers that are clearly wrong, incorrect, or appear unfit until you cannot eliminate anymore.

- Another tip here is to look out for vague answers. Avoid vague answers and if you spot one, eliminate it!

- **The true-false test.**
- Treat each option as a true-false question and choose the option that is the 'most true'.

- **Trust your common sense!**
- Even if you're not 100% sure, knowing that you have studied rigorously and have gained a good knowledge of the content, it is often better to trust your instinct rather than risk running out of time.

- Even more than instinct, try and use your common sense and re-read the question again to see whether there is a key aspect you have overlooked at first sight!

- Another strategy that you can use is to read the question, answer the question and pick the option that most closely matches your answer.

- **Look for similar options.**

- Looking for the odd answer is a test strategy that can also prove very useful. See whether the three similar options are related to a completely different topic and use the method of elimination or/and the true-false test to narrow down your correct answer.

- **Look for opposite/echo options.**
- If two questions are the opposite of one another, chances are that one of them is correct.

Section 17: Final Notes

I'd like to take this opportunity to thank you for purchasing this book. I hope you now have a solid foundation, and that this guide has helped you equip yourself with the knowledge for achieving success with the lab value questions in the NCLEX, and throughout your nursing career.

My final piece of advice - no matter how diligent you are in your studies, your best learning will come from proactively practicing questions over and over again. I recommend revisiting the questions you have found difficult to constantly refresh and build on your knowledge as you progress.

I sincerely wish you the best of luck in your nursing career.

Best wishes,

Eva Regan